Getting Back to the Happy Place

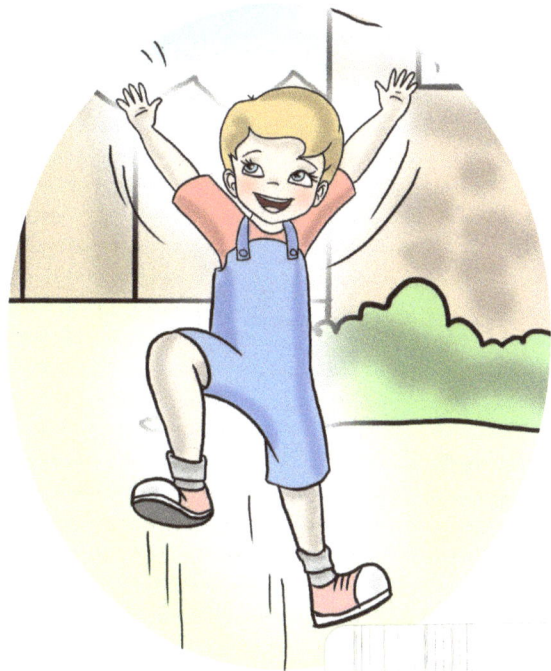

by

Josh Rubin
Known as "Pops" by his Grandkids

Mazo Publishers

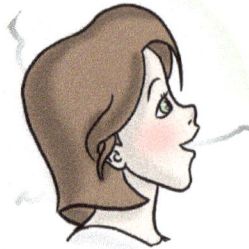
Mom

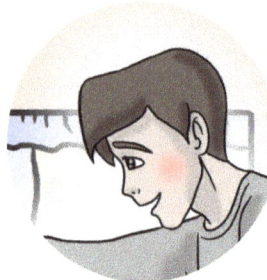
Dad

Getting Back To The Happy Place
ISBN: 978-1-956381-07-8
Josh (Yehoshua) Rubin – Copyright © 2022
Also available in Hebrew

Author
Josh (Yehoshua) Rubin
is a Life Coach and Therapist with a Masters in Counseling.
He is available for coaching and counseling sessions.

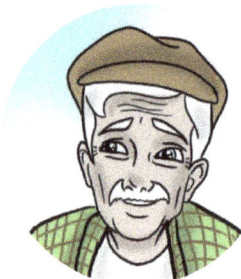
Pops

Contact Josh Rubin
WhatsApp: +972-504-259-191
Israel number: 0504-259-191
Email: yehoshuarubin@gmail.com

M

Mazo Publishers
Chaim Mazo, Publisher
www.mazopublishers.com
chaim@mazopublishers.com

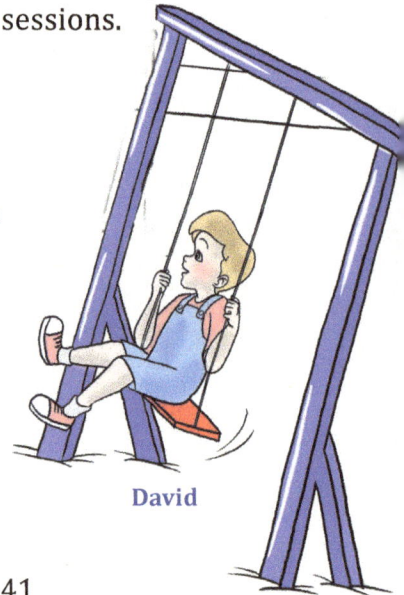
David

Editor – Shoshana Lepon
Illustrator – Shira Peled: 0559-183-141

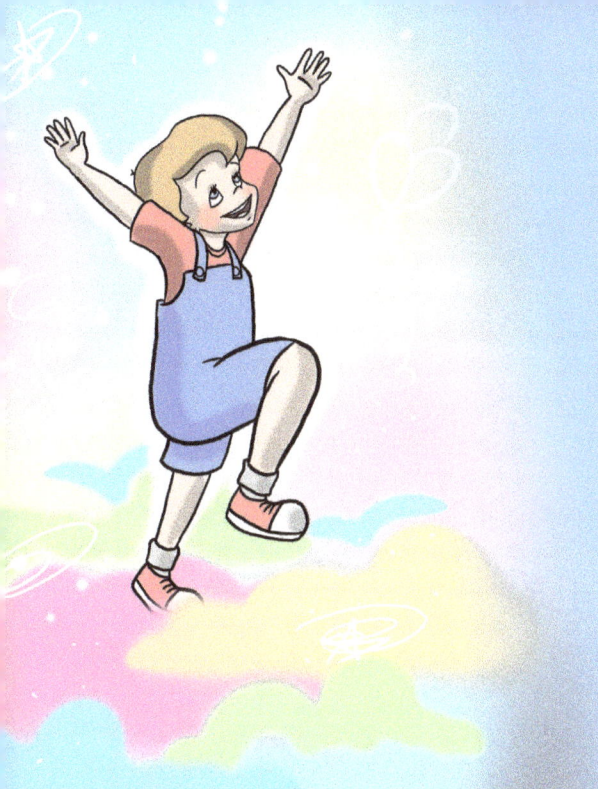

David likes to be in the Happy Place.

Sometimes his mom and dad come to the Happy Place with him. They play games, draw pictures together, or put on music and dance.

But sometimes David's parents are not in the Happy Place. Sometimes they yell at each other.

That's when David's stomach hurts.

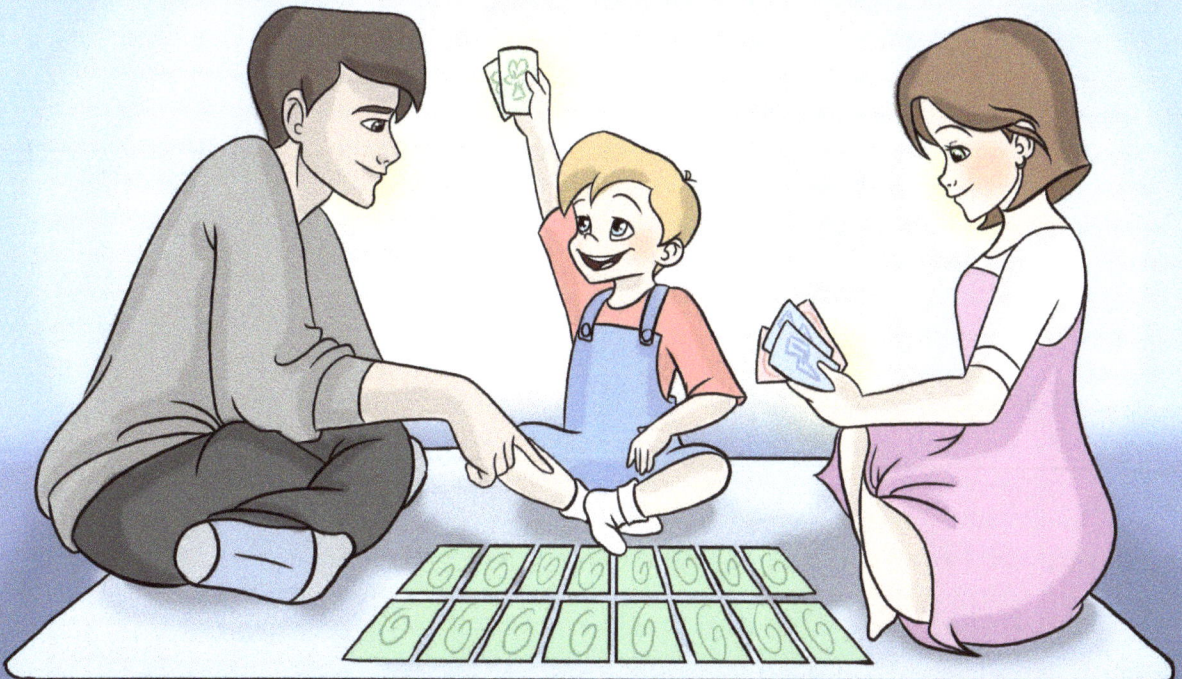

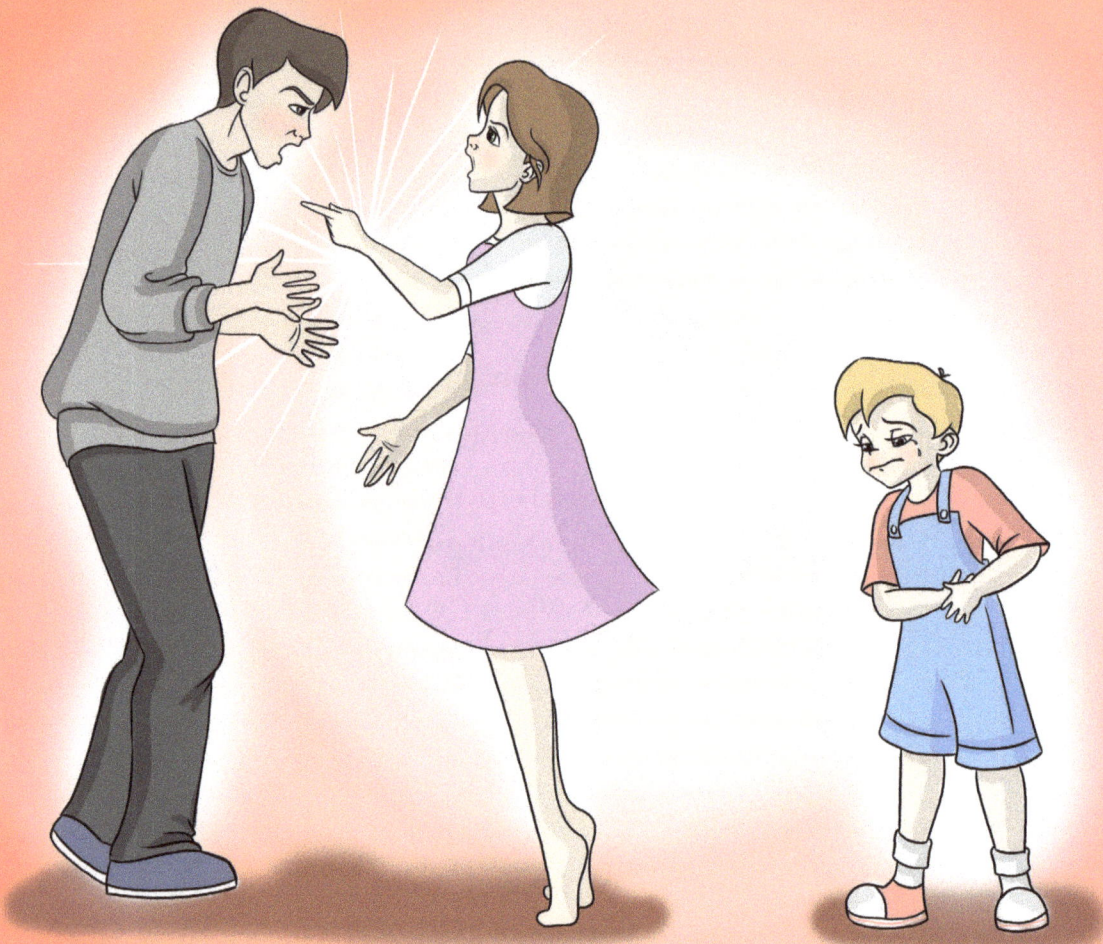

David's grandpa, Pops, told him all about the Happy Place. It's the place inside yourself, where you feel warm and good.

Pops said that when we are in the Happy Place, we smile, have lots of energy, and we can even talk instead of yelling.

Pops knows that when his parents yell at each other, David's tummy hurts.

Pops told him, "David, when your parents yell, remember the happy place. This is the place where anything is possible and then your stomach will not hurt anymore."

But right now, David feels bad and doesn't know what to do.

He wonders, "Will we ever get back to the Happy Place?"

Every week Pops and David go for a walk.

The doorbell rings and David runs to the door. "It's Pops!" he calls out and then gives Pops a big hug.

Pops laughs, "Looks like someone is ready to go."

"I sure am," says David. "I even have a water bottle."

Pops and David wave to Mom and Dad and they head out.

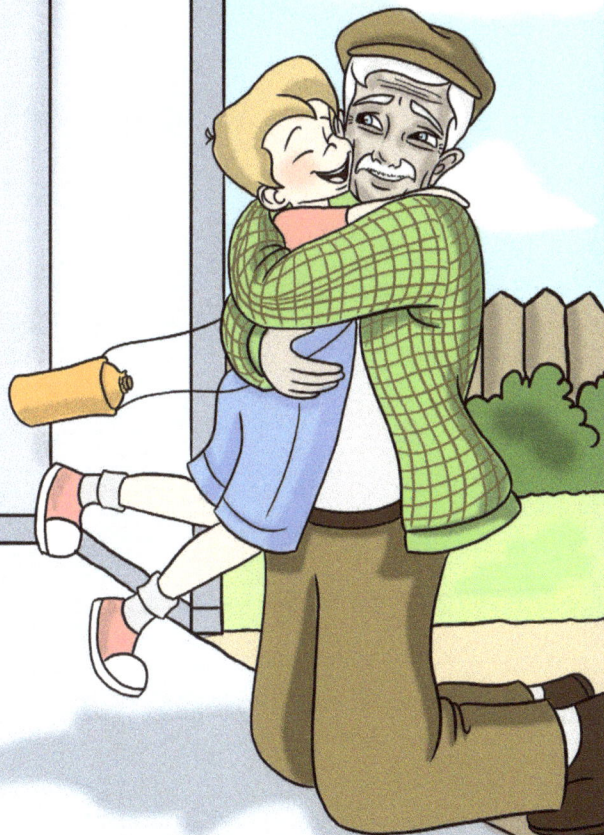

It is springtime, and David's backyard is green and flowering.

His backyard leads to his favorite playground with the red slide. David knows that on their walk they will walk through the forest with the tall pine trees, until they reach their special place on top of the hill, from where they can see the entire valley.

While holding Pops' hand, David thinks to himself: "Pops has such warm hands."

After walking for a while, Pops turns to David and asks, "So how are you doing today?"

David shrugs, "Ok, I guess."

"When I knocked on the door, I heard your parents fighting."

"Yeah, and it makes my stomach hurt when they fight."

Pops gently put his hand on David's shoulder and said, "My stomach also hurts when I hear people fighting."

"I wish my parents spent more time in the Happy Place. They never yell when they're in the Happy Place. I am scared that we will not find the way back to the Happy Place."

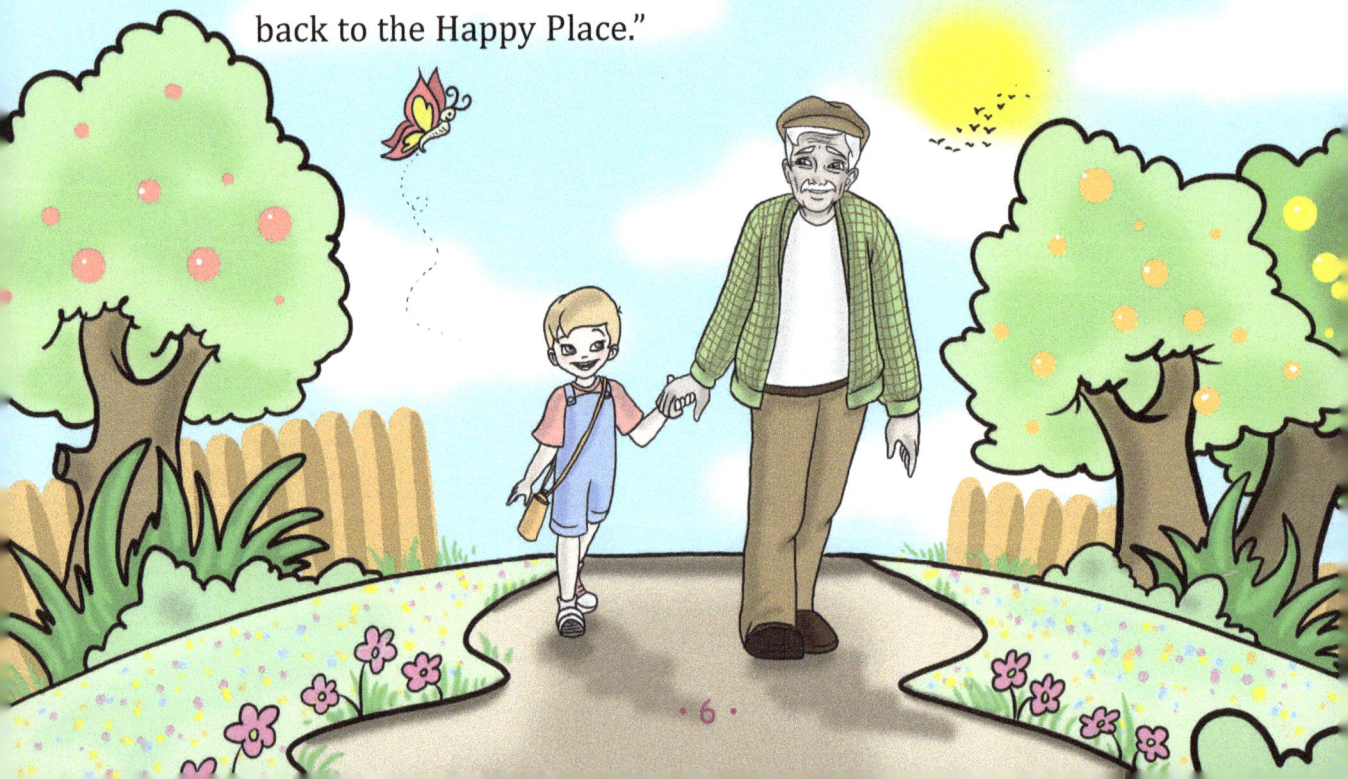

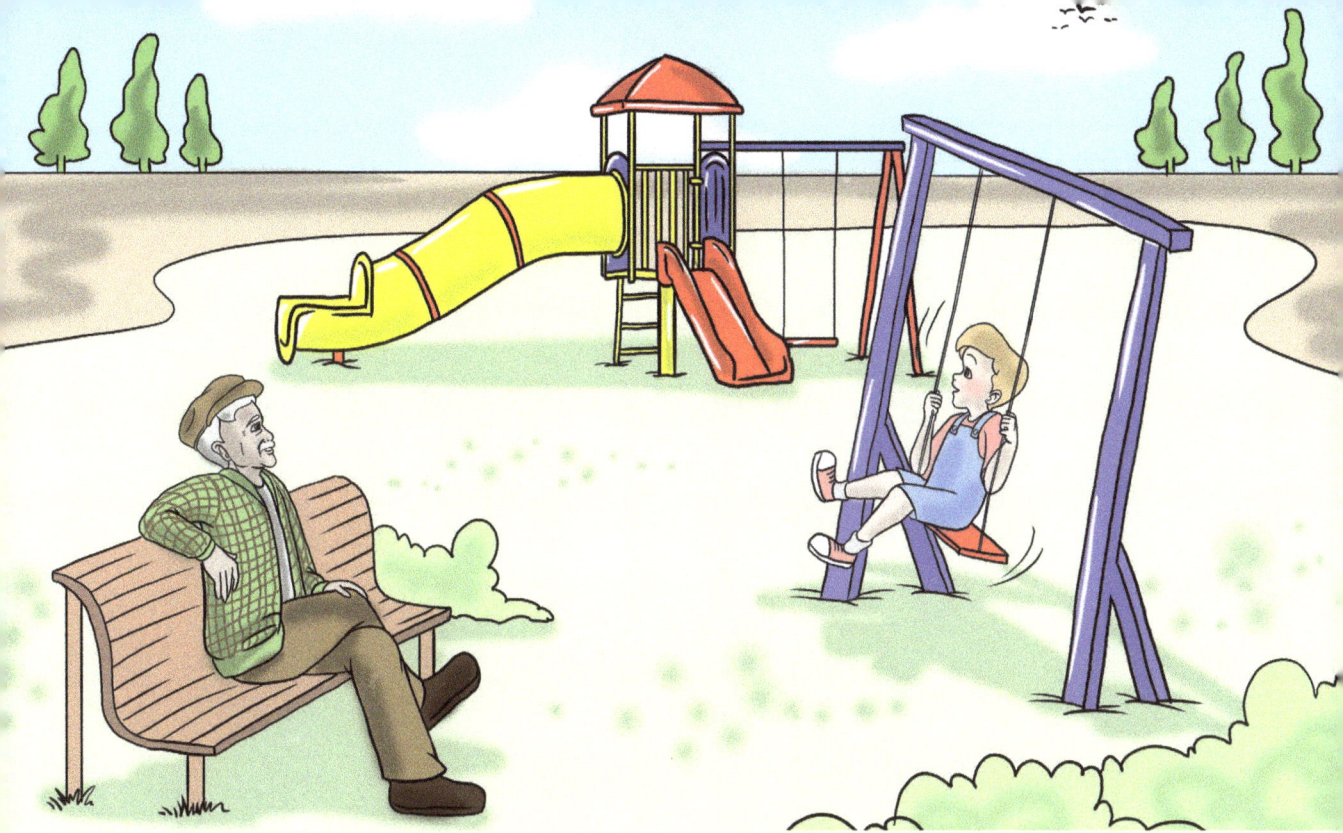

Pops listens and his eyes look sad, but he doesn't say a word.

Sometimes Pops gets quiet because he's thinking. Pops likes to think before he speaks.

Finally Pops says, "Time to play."

Pops watches David climb up on the swing, lean back and pump his legs in the air. Then to the climbing tower and down the big slide.

When David runs back to the bench, Pops asks him, "Does your stomach still hurt?"

"No, it doesn't!" David says in surprise.

"Do you know why?"

David isn't sure. He asks, "Is it because I'm back in my Happy Place?"

"Exactly," Pops answers with a smile. "Doing something fun takes you to your Happy Place!"

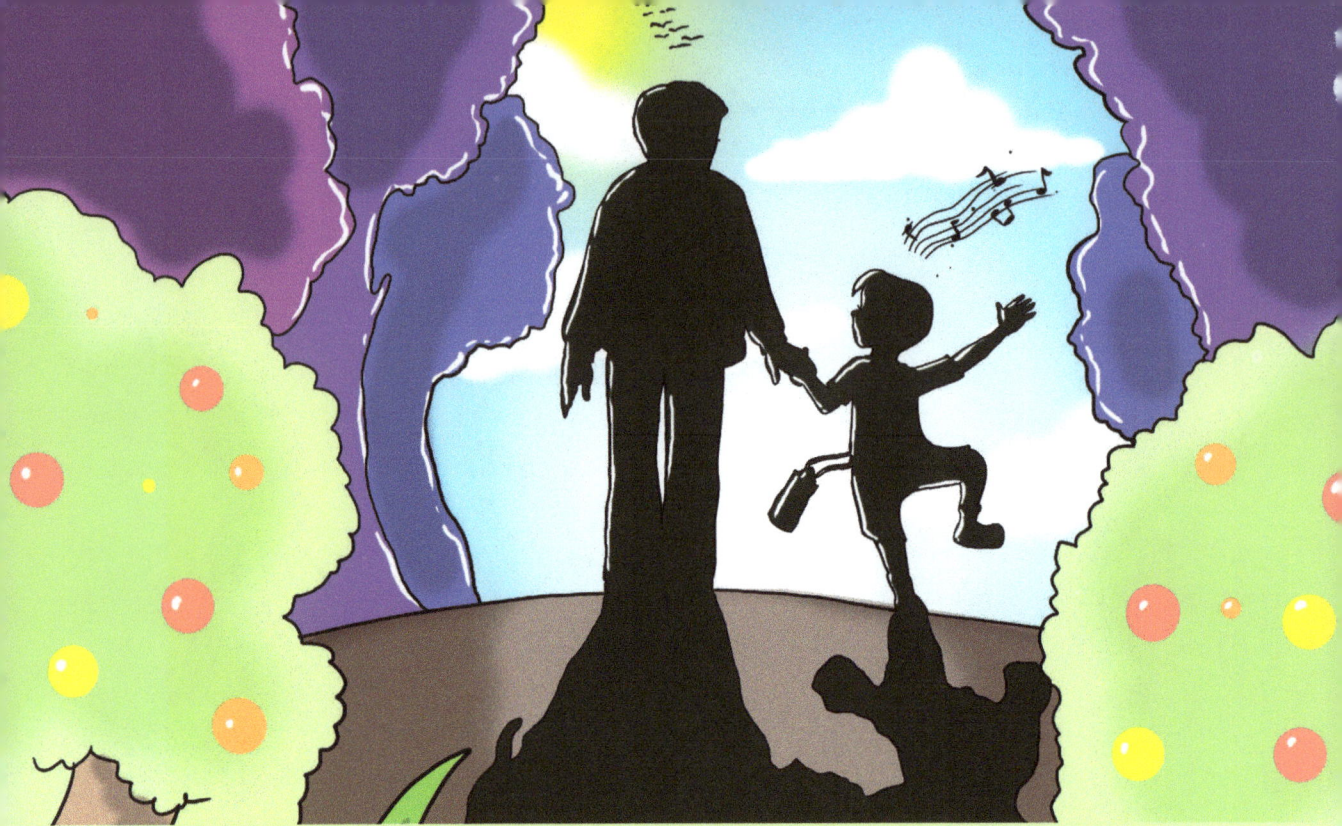

From the playground they follow the path through the forest with the tall trees. As they walk, Pops starts to sing their favorite song, to the tune of "Twinkle, Twinkle Little Star".

> *"Walking and playing*
>
> *Is so much fun,*
>
> *I feel so happy*
>
> *Walking here with you."*

Pops and David keep singing the words over and over. Sometimes they just have fun and just hum.

Pops asks, "David, tell me something … When you were singing, did you think about all the things that are bothering you?"

"No, I didn't, Pops."

"Well, singing also takes us back to the Happy Place. And then we may feel good enough to share what's bothering us."

"Why does being in our Happy Place make it easier to share?" asks David.

"Because, when we are sad, we have a heavy feeling in our body. We feel far away from people and just want to be alone," Pops explains.

"But when we're happy, the heavy feeling goes away, and we feel full of energy! We want to run around and be with people. And then it's easier to tell them what's bothering us."

"You mean like when my parents are shouting?"

"Yes, like that."

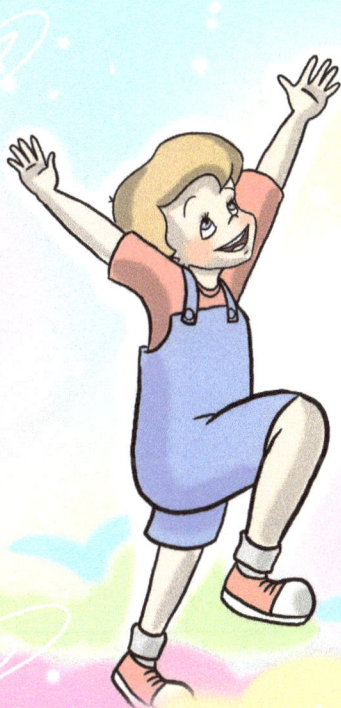

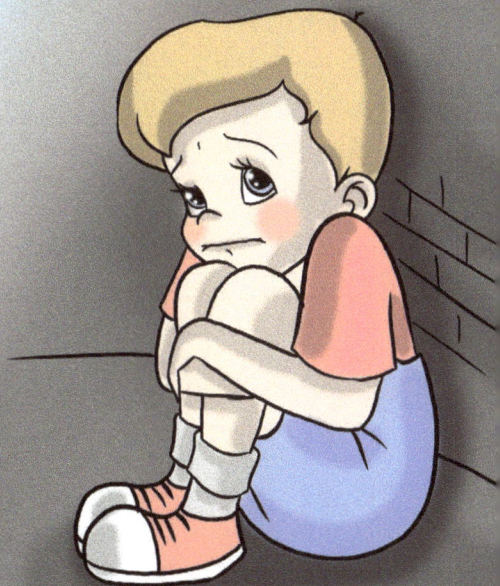

Pops and David continue walking, singing and laughing. The birds chirping in the tall trees seem to echo their happy mood. Pops and David enjoy the gentle breeze that blows through the trees. And it seems that the birds enjoy the breeze, too.

When they leave the forest, David starts to run to the top of the hill. As always, he is rewarded with the amazing view of the valley.

Pops catches up to David and sits himself down on the bench. David hears Pops breathing hard.

Pops says, "Let's sit for a minute." It is easier to relax in such a quiet and beautiful place. David's happy to sit, and finds himself breathing slower. He notices how peaceful he feels. Almost without thinking about it, David rests his head against Pops. Then he feels Pops putting his arm around his shoulders.

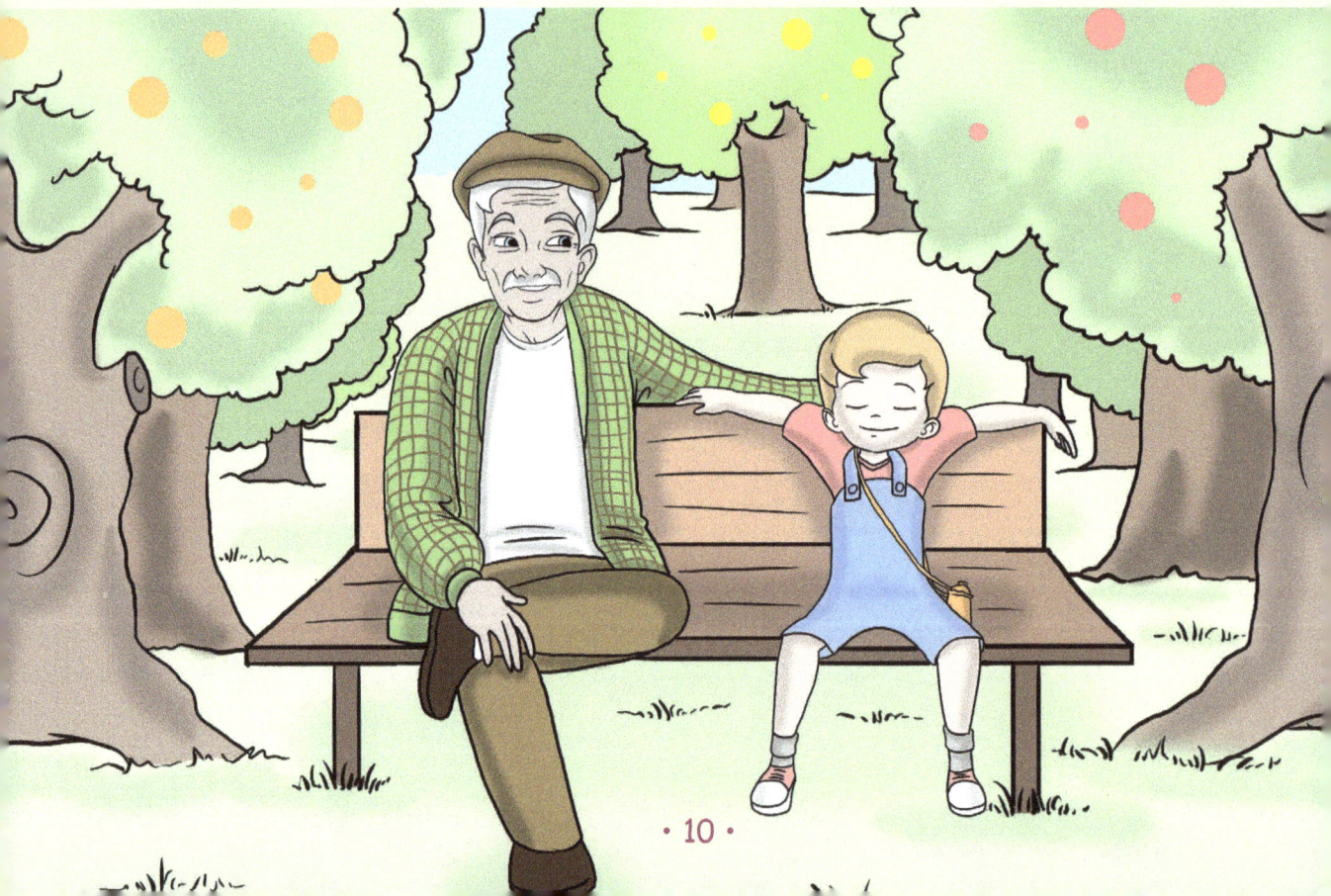

Pops says, "David, there is another way to go to our Happy Place."

"You mean something different from playing and singing?" David asks.

"Yes," Pops answers. "Relaxing is another way to go back to the Happy Place inside ourselves."

Curious, David asks, "How do you do that?"

"Well, the first step is to sit and relax like you just did. Also, choosing a quiet place outside makes it easier to relax."

"But Pops, I'm already sitting!" laughs David.

"Yes, you're sitting, but are you relaxed?"

"Relaxed?"

"Yes. Relaxing is another way to get back to the Happy Place."

"How do you do it?"

"You need to sit still, breathe slowly and see how beautiful everything is around you. You become more and more quiet, and it feels like your insides are slowing down. Want to try?"

"Ok."

Breathing slowly and smelling the trees, Pops asks David, "Are you relaxing?"

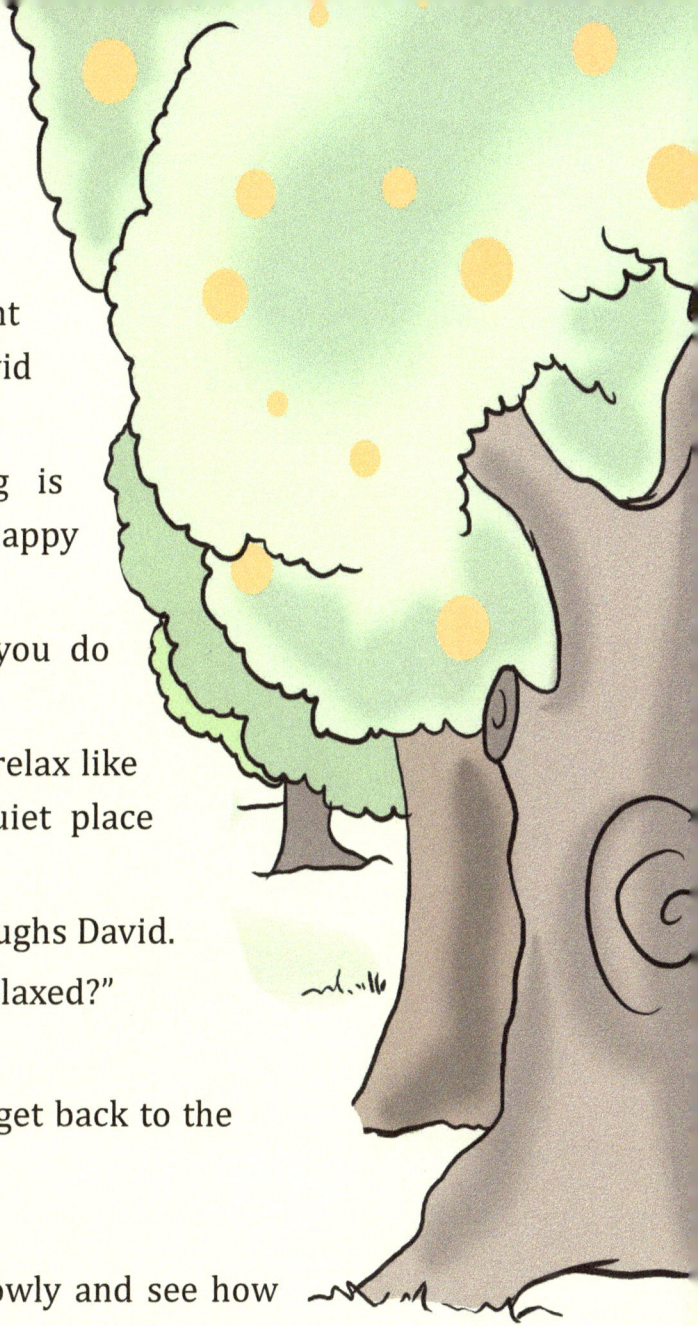

"No," sighs David. "Even though I stopped talking, I keep thinking about the things that bother me."

"Let's try again. This time, look at the sky. At the clouds. See how the clouds gently drift from one side of the sky to the other, until they vanish."

It was quiet while they looked at the clouds gently drifting away.

"Do you see?"

"Yes," whispers David.

"Ok," says Pops. "Now breathe slowly and imagine that each cloud is holding something that bothers you. When the cloud floats away, see your troubles floating away with it. No more worries!"

Pops and David lean back, take slow, deep breaths and watch the clouds drifting above them. This time, David thinks of what's bothering him and drops it into a cloud. He follows the cloud as it slowly drifts out of sight.

"How did you learn to do that, Pops?" David wonders.

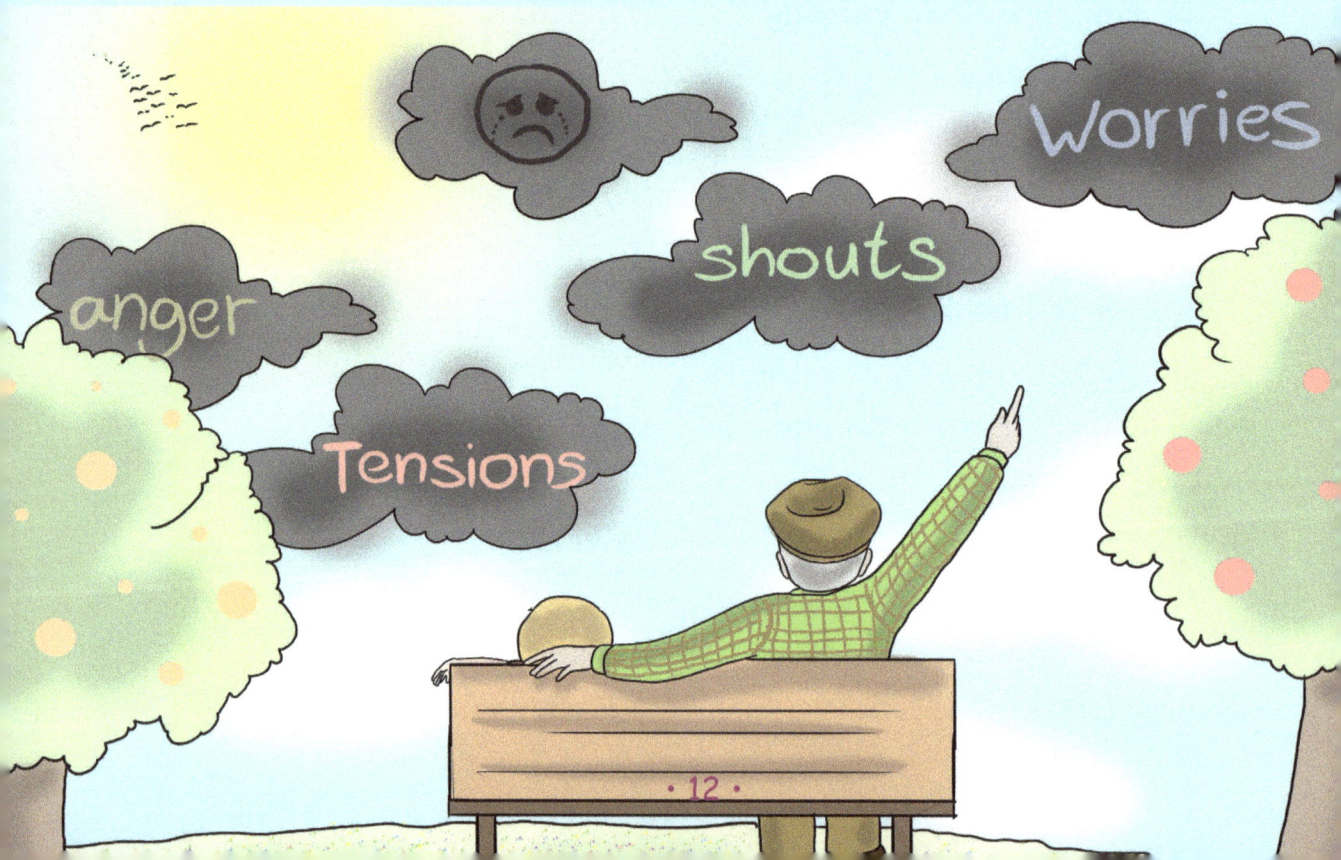

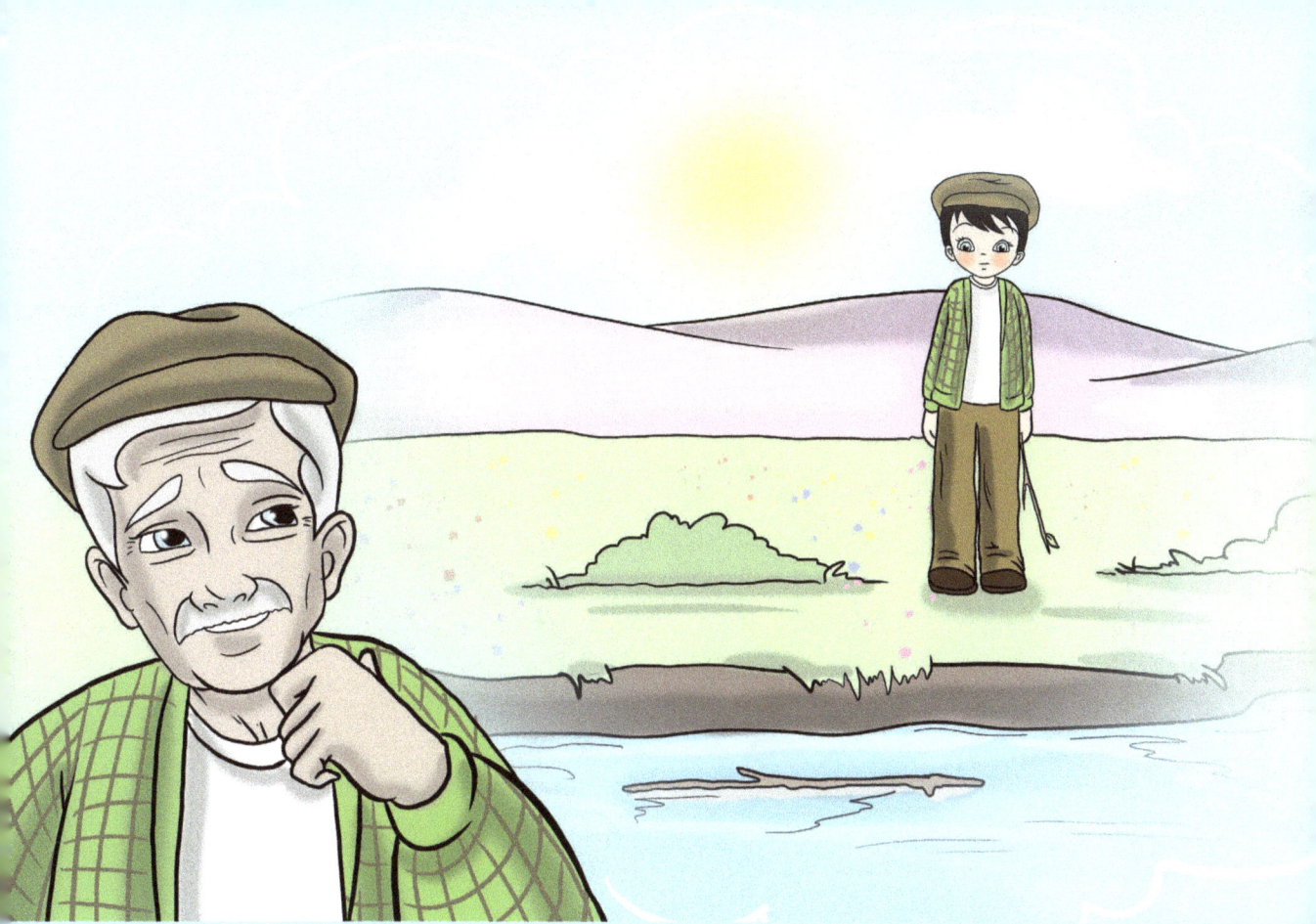

Pops looks at David, remembering a story to tell him.

"When I was little, I'd sometimes have a bad day at school. But by the time I got home, I would feel better.

"I'd stop by a creek, throw in a branch and watch it slowly float down the stream. My dad told me that watching the branches float away also helps my bad feelings float away.

"Watching the clouds in the sky does the same thing ... It helps us let go of our bad thoughts."

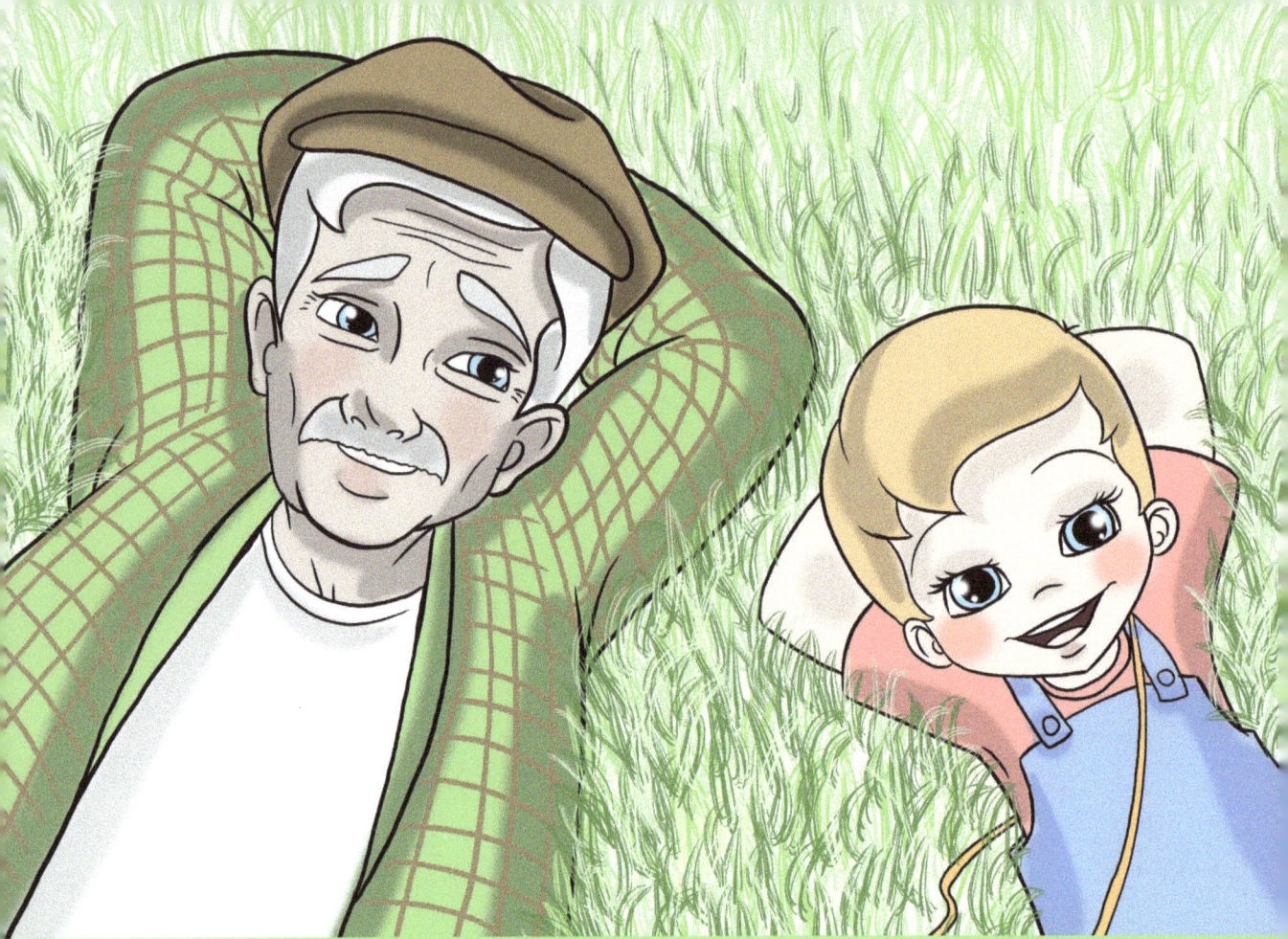

Laying on the grass and staring up at the clouds, Pops says, "Sometimes we forget about our Happy Place. And we forget how to get there. But with playing, singing and relaxing, we can always find our way back. Do you think you can do that, David?"

David smiles up at his grandfather.

"Pops," he says, "I think I can."

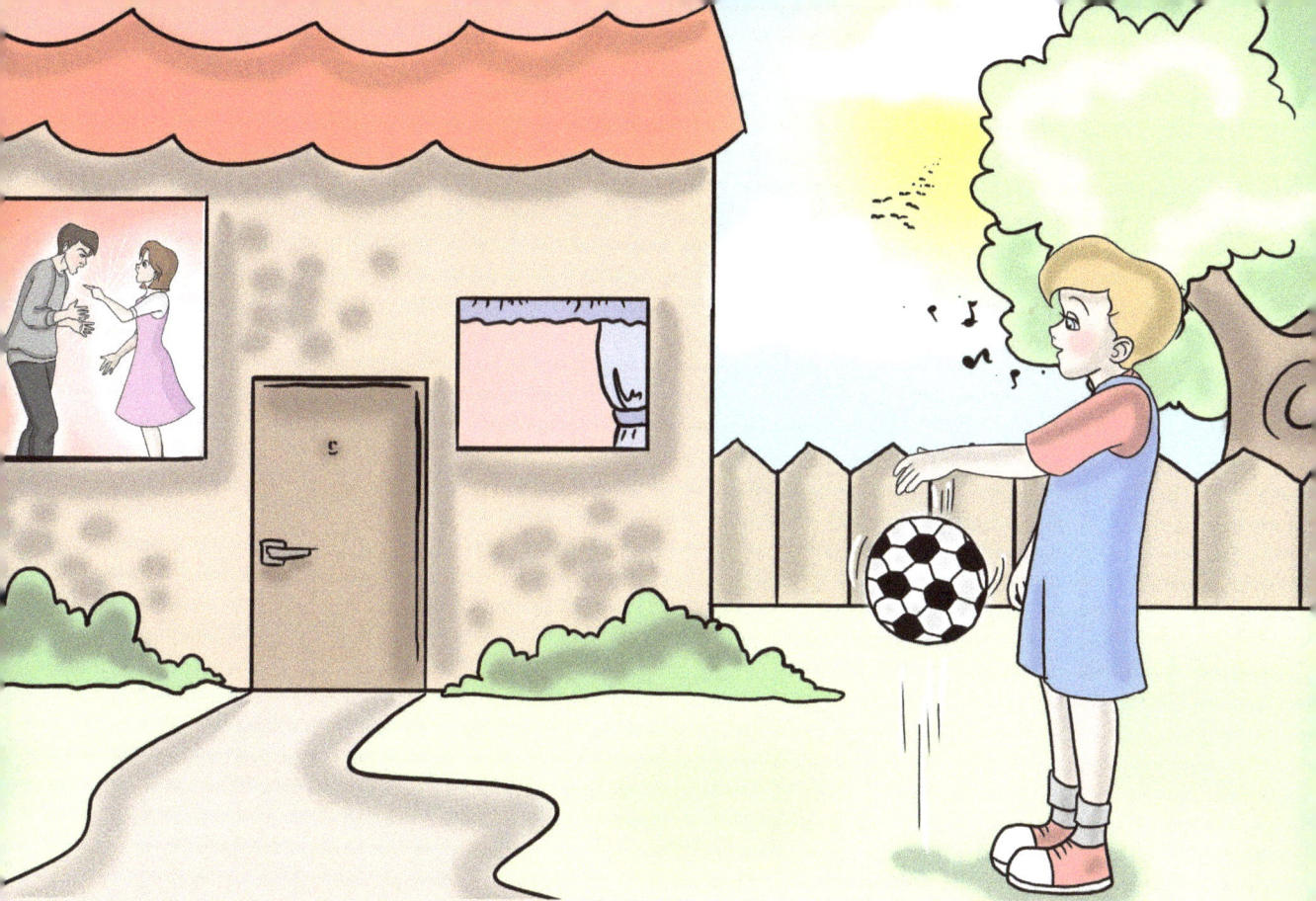

As the days go by, David notices how much better he feels. When he plays, sings or just looks up at the clouds, his stomach stops hurting. He likes to be in the Happy Place.

One day, David hears his parents yelling and feels his stomach getting tight.

This time, he runs outside and kicks a ball. As he plays, he sings the song that Pops taught him, to the tune of "Twinkle, Twinkle, Little Star".

"Walking and playing
Is so much fun,
I feel so happy
Walking here with you."

David keeps repeating the song again and again, remembering everything Pops taught him. Soon he feels how wonderful it is to be outside and play.

David feels happy. Once again, he finds the Happy Place.

"Walking and playing
Is so much fun,
I feel so happy
Walking here with you."

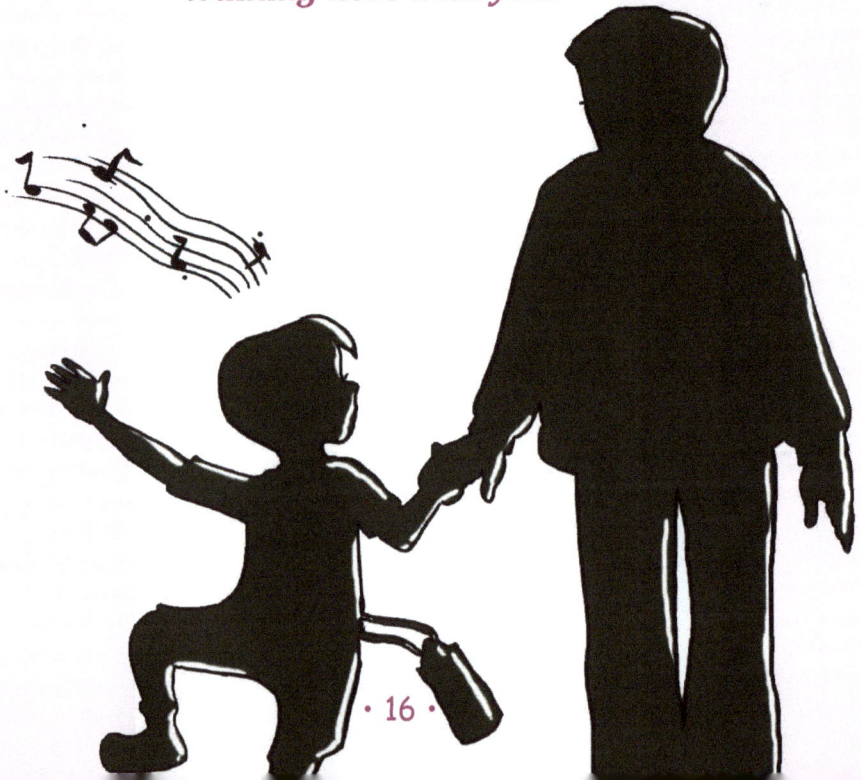

"Walking and playing
Is so much fun,
I feel so happy
Walking here with you."

"Walking and playing
Is so much fun,
I feel so happy
Walking here with you."

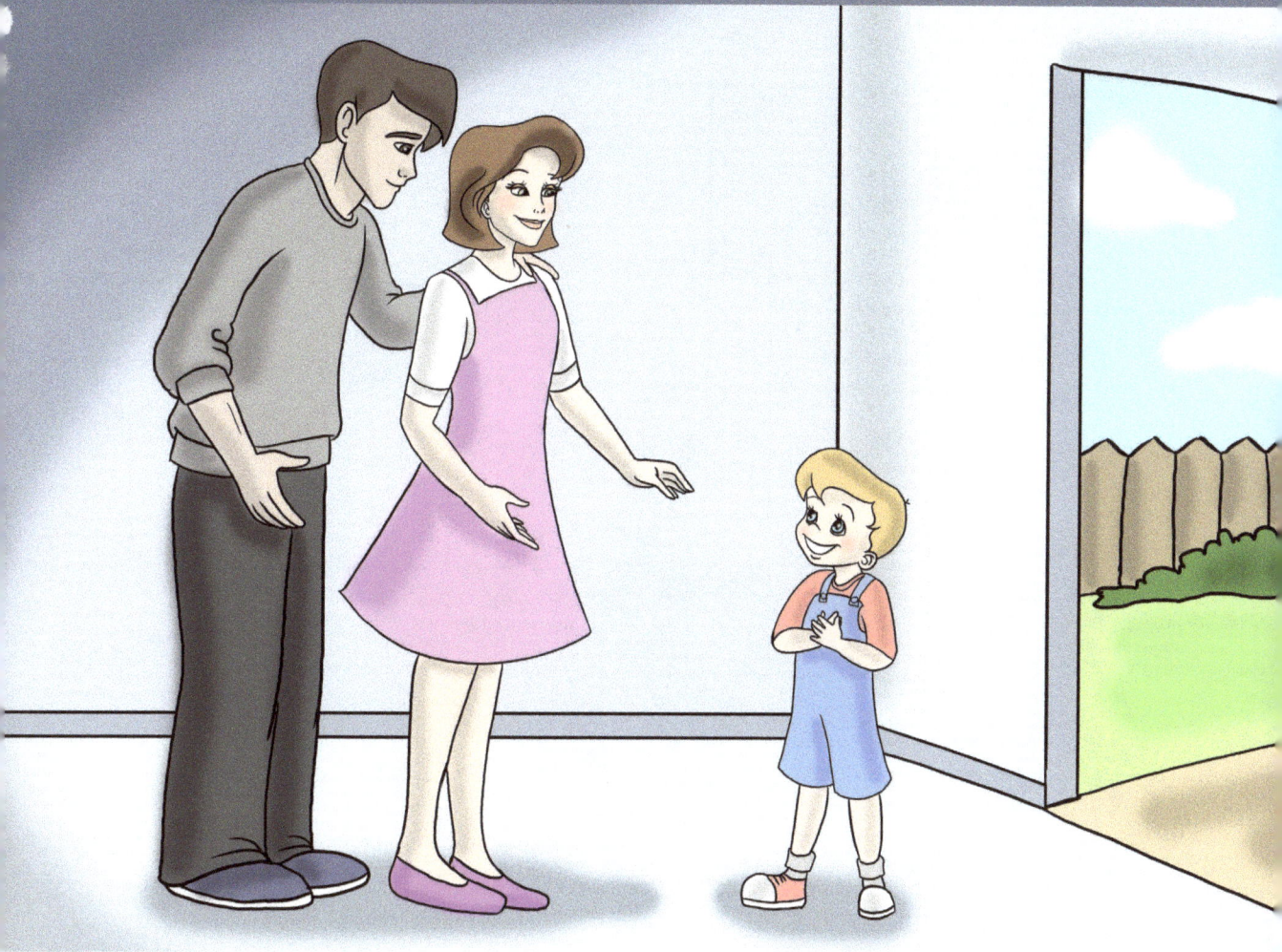

David wonders if his parents would like to go to the Happy Place with him. He slowly opens the front door and waits for his parents to see him.

"Hi Mom. Hi Dad," he says. "It scares me when you yell at each other. Pops taught me how to get to the Happy Place. Could we all go there together?"

His parents stand there staring at each other. Finally, Mom says, "I remember the Happy Place from when I was little. Pops used to take me there when we went on walks. It's a good place to go to."

Dad says, "You're right. It's been a while since I have been in my Happy Place."

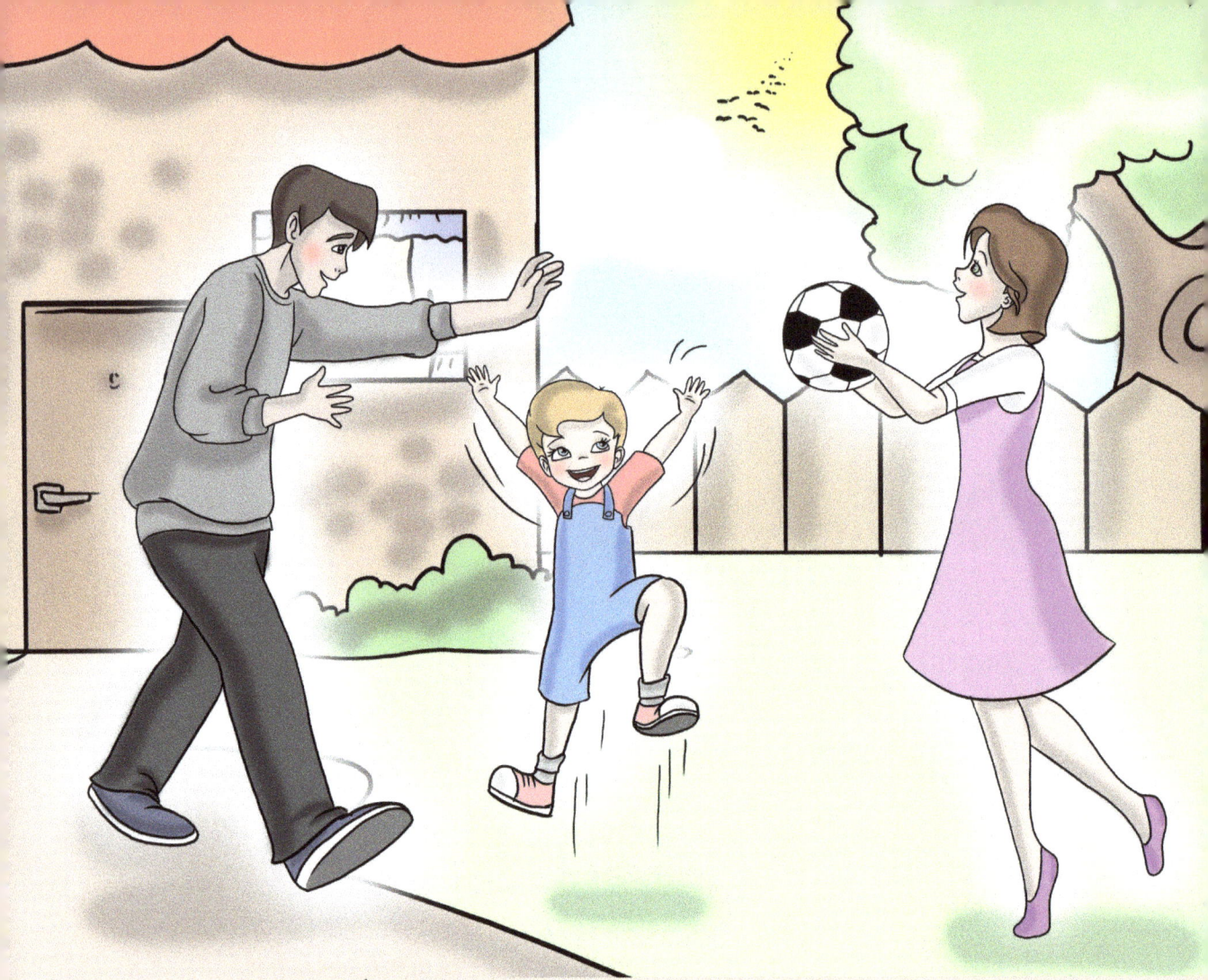

So David and his parents go into the front yard.

David picks up his ball. "I throw to Mom, Mom throws to Dad and Dad throws to me."

They play for a long time, tossing the ball back and forth and laughing when they miss.

"Hey!" Dad says, "This is great! We should go to the Happy Place more often."

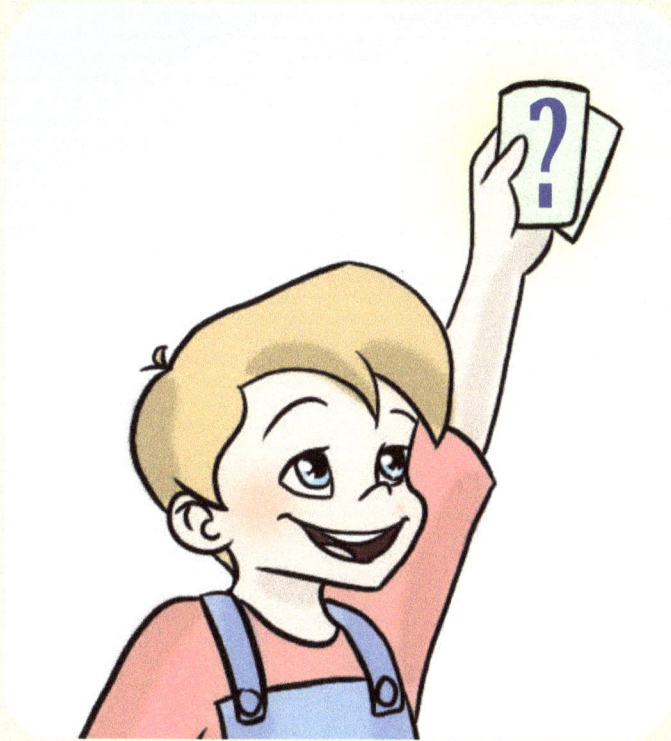

Questions for Discussion

- What helps you get to the Happy Place?

- What happens at home or at school that makes you leave the Happy Place?

- What reminds you of how to get back to the Happy Place?

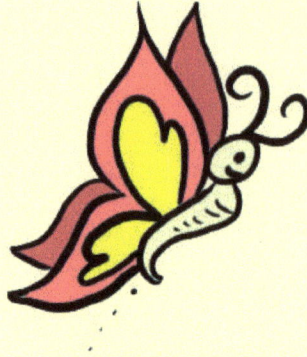

Josh (Yehoshua) Rubin, the author of this book,
is a Life Coach and Therapist with a Masters in Counseling.
He is available for coaching and counseling sessions.

Contact Josh Rubin
WhatsApp: +972-504-259-191
Israel number: 0504-259-191
Email: yehoshuarubin@gmail.com

www.ingramcontent.com/pod-product-compliance
Lightning Source LLC
Chambersburg PA
CBHW041431040426
42445CB00020B/1985